SWOLLEN GLANDS

A Comprehensive Strategy for the Wellness of Enlarged Gland: Maintaining a Lymphatic System in Good Working Order

CHAD BRUNO

Table of Contents

Introductory

Lymph node enlargement is medically referred to as swollen glands or lymphadenopathy. The immune system relies heavily on the lymphatic system, which includes the tiny bean-shaped structures known as lymph nodes. White blood cells are housed in these nodes and aid in the fight against infections while also filtering lymph fluid.

When the lymph nodes swell, it's usually because the body is reacting to an infection, an injury, or some other health problem. When the lymph nodes swell, it's usually a sign that the body's immune system is hard at work trying to rid itself of whatever's causing the issue. Some frequent triggers for gland swelling are:

1. One of the most prevalent causes of enlarged lymph nodes is infection. Lymph nodes in the area may expand as a result of an immune response to a bacterial, viral, or fungal infection. An infection in the throat, for instance, may cause lymph nodes in the neck to swell.

2. Lymph nodes can swell due to the activation of the immune system in response to chronic inflammation, which can occur in autoimmune illnesses and other inflammatory conditions.

3. Swollen lymph nodes may be a symptom of cancer, including lymphoma and other forms of metastatic disease. Lymph node enlargement is a potential side effect of cancer cell metastasis.

4. Other medical diseases: Allergies, responses to drugs, and systemic disorders are some other examples of non-infectious and non-cancerous conditions that can induce swollen glands.

Causes of swollen glands can sometimes be deduced from their location and the symptoms they bring with them. If you have swollen glands that won't go away or are otherwise difficult to explain, you should see a doctor right once so they can establish the source and prescribe therapy.

CHAPTER ONE
Glands: Structure and Role in the Body

In the body, glands are specialized organs or tissues that exude compounds vital to the body's proper functioning. Exocrine glands and endocrine glands are the two most common types, and they serve different purposes in the body.

1. Glandula Exocrine:

• **Structure:** the secreted compounds from exocrine glands go through ducts, which are tiny channels or tubes. These ducts may lead either to the skin or inside organs.

- **Function:** Exocrine glands discharge their products, such as enzymes, mucus, perspiration, and digestive juices, into ducts that deliver these substances to specified target locations. perspiration glands emit perspiration onto the skin's surface to cool the body down, and salivary glands release saliva into the mouth via ducts.

2. Lymph Nodes:

Because of their structure, endocrine glands do not have ducts and instead inject their hormones and other secretions straight into the circulatory system. Many people use the term "ductless" to describe these glands.

Hormones, chemical messengers that govern development, metabolism, and homeostasis, are produced and secreted by the endocrine glands. The bloodstream transports hormones all across the body to the cells and organs they're meant to affect. The pituitary gland, the thyroid gland, and the adrenal glands are all examples of endocrine glands.

Some examples of glands and the tasks they perform are as follows:

1. **Salivary Glands:** Exocrine glands that secrete saliva, an enzyme-rich fluid that aids digestion.

2. The pancreas is a multifunctional organ that controls blood sugar levels by secreting the hormones insulin and glucagon, as well as producing digestive enzymes as an exocrine function.

3. **Thyroid Gland:** Endocrine gland responsible for producing growth and metabolism-regulating hormones.

4. The adrenal glands are a pair of endocrine glands that secrete stress

hormones like adrenaline and the related hormone cortisol.

5. **Pituitary gland:** this endocrine gland, also known as the "master gland," governs many different physiological processes and regulates the activity of other endocrine glands.

6. Perspiration glands are exocrine glands that secrete perspiration to cool the body down when it gets too hot.

7. Milk is produced by the mammary glands, which are exocrine glands in the breast tissue of females.

8. Glands located on the surface of the body that produce sebum, an oily material used to moisturize the skin and hair.

The appropriate functioning of glands is vital for maintaining homeostasis and regulating many body processes. Hormonal imbalances, metabolic abnormalities, and other medical problems can result from damage to or disease of the glands. Therefore, it is necessary for both medical experts and laypeople to have an awareness of the architecture and function of glands.

Typical Roots of Gland Swelling

Lymphadenopathy, the medical term for swollen glands, can result from a number of different conditions. The lymphatic system includes the lymph nodes, which can swell in response to a number of stimuli, infection being the most prevalent. Some common triggers for gland enlargement include:

1. Infections:

Swollen lymph nodes may be the result of a bacterial infection, such as a streptococcal throat infection, tuberculosis, or an STD.

Lymph nodes may expand as a result of viral illnesses such as the common cold, influenza, mononucleosis, and HIV.

Lymphadenopathy can be brought on by o Fungal Infections like Histoplasmosis or Coccidioidomycosis.

2. Symptoms of Inflammation:

Inflammation caused by autoimmune diseases such as rheumatoid arthritis, systemic lupus erythematosus, and Sjögren's syndrome can cause enlarged lymph nodes.

Abdominal lymph node enlargement is a symptom of inflammatory bowel illness, which includes Crohn's disease and ulcerative colitis.

Lymph nodes are just one of many organs that can be affected by sarcoidosis, an inflammatory illness.

3. Cancer:

Lymphoma: Lymphoma is a malignancy of the lymphatic system and can cause the lymph nodes to grow.

Swollen lymph nodes can be a symptom of metastatic cancer,

which has migrated to the lymph nodes from another section of the body.

• **Leukemia:** Lymphadenopathy is a symptom of several forms of leukemia.

4. Reactions to Medications:

Swollen lymph nodes are a common side effect of an adverse reaction to certain drugs.

The lymph nodes may swell as a result of an allergic reaction to an allergen or an insect bite.

5. Oral and Dental Problems:

• Swollen lymph nodes, including those in the neck, have been linked to dental infections, abscesses, and other oral infections.

6. Diseases of the Immune System:

• Disorders that impact the immune system, such HIV/AIDS, can lead to persistent lymph node enlargement.

7. Different Reasons:

• Bartonella henselae infection, also known as "cat scratch disease," is spread through a cat's scratch or bite.

Kawasaki disease is an uncommon illness that predominantly affects kids and is characterized by inflammation of the lymph nodes and blood vessels.

The precise location of the swollen glands and the symptoms that accompany them can be quite helpful in making a diagnosis. Swollen glands are a common immune system reaction to infection, and they often go away once the infection is treated. However, if your glands are continuously enlarged without an evident explanation or if they are accompanied by other troubling symptoms, you should consult a doctor to evaluate the cause and the best course of therapy.

CHAPTER TWO
Diagnosis and Manifestations

Swollen glands (lymphadenopathy) can present with a wide range of symptoms, depending on the etiology, lymph node location, and duration of the swelling. The following are some of the most often reported signs of enlarged lymph nodes:

1. Lymph Node Enlargement: you may feel a lump or bump under your skin, which may be very little or fairly substantial.

2. Tenderness or Pain: Swollen lymph nodes can be uncomfortable or painful to the touch, especially when squeezed or manipulated.

3. Skin redness and warmth: the skin above the afflicted lymph nodes may become red and warm.

4. Swollen glands and fever are common symptoms of bacterial and viral infections.

5. Fatigue, loss of appetite, night sweats, and weight loss are all examples of general symptoms that can arise from a variety of different conditions.

6. Location-specific symptoms: Swollen glands in distinct locations of the body might lead to region-specific symptoms. A sore throat could be the result of swollen lymph nodes in the neck, while groin swelling could make walking painful.

Swollen glands require a comprehensive medical evaluation, which may consist of the following procedures:

1. Your doctor will inquire about your current health, past illnesses, and any new infections. Other symptoms, recent travel, and possible exposure to infectious agents may also be discussed.

2. The doctor will perform a physical check to determine the reason of the swelling in your lymph nodes by taking a look at your overall health and noting any abnormalities.

3. Analytical Procedures:

• Blood tests: These can be used to look for indicators of illness, such as infection, inflammation, or even HIV.

• **Biopsy:** if the swelling of a lymph node cannot be explained by other factors, a tissue sample may be taken and examined under a microscope. This is commonly done when there is a lack of explanation for lymphadenopathy's persistence.

4. Ultrasound, computed tomography (CT), and magnetic resonance imaging (MRI) scans are examples of imaging studies that may be used to observe the lymph nodes and adjacent tissues, as well as to detect any abnormalities.

5. Cultures and serological tests are two examples of the types of diagnostic procedures that may be used to determine whether bacteria, viruses, or other pathogens are present in an infectious disease patient.

6. Further Specialist review: Depending on the first assessment and test results, you may be sent to a specialist, such as an infectious disease specialist, oncologist, or rheumatologist, for a more in-depth review and care.

The specifics of the diagnostic procedure will be determined by the patient's symptoms, medical history, and the suspected etiology of the enlarged glands. It's vital to visit a healthcare practitioner if you suffer chronic or severe symptoms or have concerns about swollen glands, as a timely and precise diagnosis is essential for optimal treatment.

Alternative Treatments

Lymphadenopathy is the medical term for swollen glands, and its therapy is condition specific. Sometimes, when the underlying problem improves, the swollen glands will go away on their own because they are a natural immune reaction to infection. However, if your swollen glands are the result of something more serious or persistent, you may need to seek out specialized care. Some frequent methods of treatment are as follows:

1. Getting to the Root of the Problem:

Infections: Antibiotics may be recommended if the enlarged glands are caused by bacteria. Antibiotics are ineffective against viruses, thus supportive care is the standard treatment.

Anti-inflammatory pharmaceuticals, disease-modifying therapies, and other condition-specific treatments may be used for the management of inflammatory disorders.

When lymph node swelling is due to cancer, treatment options include removal of the affected lymph nodes, chemotherapy, radiation therapy, immunotherapy, or a combination of these methods.

2. Relieving Symptoms:

Swollen glands can cause pain and discomfort, which can be treated with over-the-counter pain medicines such acetaminophen or ibuprofen.

• Warm Compresses: Applying warm compresses to the afflicted area may help relieve pain and facilitate drainage.

3. Keeping tabs and looking over things:

If a doctor suspects that your swollen glands are due to anything small that will clear up on its own, such a recent infection, he or she may decide to keep an eye on them. If there is no improvement or if the symptoms increase, additional assessment may be recommended.

4. Interventions in Surgery:

When the origin of enlarged lymph nodes is unknown, a tissue sample can be obtained by a surgical procedure called a lymph node biopsy.

5. Health & Wellness at Home:

Maintaining healthy levels of hydration is essential for optimal immune function and general wellbeing.

- **Sleep:** Getting enough shut-eye helps speed recovery from infections and lessen associated discomfort.

- **Proper Diet:** A healthy diet loaded with nutrients like vitamins and minerals can help the body recover itself and strengthen the immune system.

If you have consistently swollen glands or other troubling

symptoms, it is crucial to follow the counsel of a healthcare expert for the most appropriate treatment strategy. Talking to your doctor about your personal risk factors for diseases like cancer and autoimmune disorders can help in their early detection and treatment.

Always consult a medical practitioner to establish the root cause of your swollen glands and the best course of therapy, as self-diagnosis and self-treatment may not be appropriate in many circumstances.

CHAPTER THREE
How to Avoid Gland Enlargement

Preventing swollen glands (lymphadenopathy) mostly includes maintaining excellent general health and minimizing the risk of infections and other disorders that might lead to lymph node enlargement. It's not always feasible to completely avoid getting swollen glands, but there are things you may do to lessen your chances. Some general advice on how to avoid gland swelling:

1. Wash your hands with soap and water often, especially before meals and after using the restroom, to maintain good hygiene.

To prevent the spread of germs, cover your mouth and nose when you cough or sneeze by using a tissue or your elbow.

2. Vaccinations:

A number of illnesses can cause swollen glands, so it's important to keep up with your vaccinations. If you want to know what vaccines you should get based on your age, health, and where you live, you should go to a doctor.

3. Containing Infections:

It's especially important to keep your distance from sick people when flu and cold season roll around.

- If you have a contagious illness, you should practice good hygiene to stop it from spreading.

Safe sexual behavior and the use of barrier techniques, such as condoms, can greatly lower the likelihood of contracting a STI.

4. Healthful Oral Care:

- Prevent tooth infections, which can cause swelling neck lymph nodes, by practicing proper oral hygiene with regular brushing and flossing.

5. Nutrition and Diet:

Eat a healthy, well-rounded diet full of antioxidants, vitamins, and minerals to keep your immune system in top shape.

• Drink plenty of water to keep yourself hydrated.

6. Exercising and Eating Right:

Exercise regularly; it's been shown to improve immunity and general health.

• Learn to relax in order to keep your immune system strong; stress management is essential.

7. Treatment of Allergies:

If you have allergies, it's best to avoid being around triggers as much as possible and learn how to cope with them.

Do what your doctor tells you to do if you suffer from allergies or an allergic response.

8. Precautions for Your Trip:

• If you are going to a region where infectious diseases are common, make sure to take the necessary safety measures. Consult a healthcare provider about essential immunizations and preventive measures.

9. Maintenance Exams:

Preventative treatment, screenings, and early diagnosis of health issues can all be achieved by scheduling routine visits with your healthcare professional.

Some causes of enlarged glands, such as those caused by autoimmune illnesses or genetic factors, cannot be avoided. The chance of acquiring swollen glands owing to infectious causes can be mitigated, however, by adhering to a healthy lifestyle, maintaining proper hygiene, and being careful about preventative measures. Get checked out by a doctor if your swollen glands are making you nervous, or if you have any other health problems.

Accumulation of Fluid in the Gland

Certain demographics are more likely to experience lymphadenopathy (swollen glands), and there may be demographic differences in the underlying causes and concerns. Here are some things to think about while dealing with swollen glands in vulnerable groups:

1. Children:

• Upper respiratory infections, tonsillitis, and ear infections are major causes of swollen glands in youngsters.

The mumps and the chickenpox are just two examples of viral illnesses that can cause enlarged salivary glands.

• Vaccines given to children are crucial in preventing the spread of infectious diseases that might lead to lymph node swelling.

2. Expectant Mothers:

Hormonal shifts during pregnancy might make a woman more susceptible to infection, which can lead to swollen lymph nodes in the neck, armpits, and groin.

• Mild infections or inflammatory diseases may cause swollen lymph nodes during pregnancy.

3. Senior Citizens:

• There are infectious and non-infectious causes of swollen glands in the elderly.

- Lymphoma and metastasized cancer are the most common causes of lymphadenopathy in the elderly.

As we get older, our immune systems may become less effective, leaving us more vulnerable to illness.

4. People with Weak Immune Systems

Opportunistic infections and swollen glands are more common in people with weakened immune systems, such as those who have HIV/AIDS, have received an organ transplant, or are on immunosuppressive drugs.

Lymphadenopathy is more difficult to diagnose and treat in immunocompromised patients, who typically need specific medical attention.

5. Specific Considerations for Women and Men:

A symptom of metastasis in women with breast cancer is enlargement of the lymph nodes under the arm (axillary lymph nodes).

Lymph nodes in the groin may swell in men who have testicular cancer.

6. Dangers in the Workplace:

o Contact with infectious agents, chemicals, or other possible sources of inflammation or infection may raise the risk of swollen glands in the workplace.

7. Factors Related to the Environment:

Swollen glands are more likely to occur in people who live in or visit locations where certain infections are more common, such as tuberculosis. The diagnosis and evaluation of lymphadenopathy may be affected by where the patient lives.

Since the underlying causes of swollen glands and the potential repercussions might differ greatly between special populations, prompt medical examination and therapy is essential. It's vital to see a doctor if you or a member of a high-risk group develops swollen glands or related symptoms so that you can get a proper diagnosis and the care you need. Swollen glands can have a variety of causes, so it's important to treat each patient according to his or her unique symptoms and medical history.

CHAPTER FOUR
Problems that might arise from untreated lymphedema

Depending on the underlying reason and the severity of the problem, untreated swollen glands (lymphadenopathy) can lead to a variety of consequences. In order to avoid or control further consequences, treating the underlying cause of the edema is essential. Untreated swollen glands can lead to the following consequences.

1. Disease Transmission:

A bacterial or viral infection, which may cause swollen glands, can spread through the body and cause more serious sickness if left untreated.

Streptococcal throat infections, for instance, can lead to more serious illnesses like rheumatic fever or scarlet fever if left untreated.

2. Formation of an Abscess:

• Sometimes an abscess will form as a result of a localized infection near the enlarged lymph nodes. Pustules, or abscesses, are infections that need to be drained and treated.

• **For example,** untreated dental infections can lead to abscesses in the mouth or jaw, which may impact the adjacent lymph nodes.

3. Cellulitis:

A bacterial skin infection known as cellulitis can develop if an infection of the skin or soft tissues is left untreated. Rapid dissemination of cellulitis might cause involvement of regional lymph nodes.

4. Long-Term Infections:

• If an infection isn't treated, it can persist and worsen over time. Lymphadenopathy and other systemic consequences might continue even after a chronic viral infection such as HIV or hepatitis has been treated.

5. Inflammatory disease complications:

• Swollen glands caused to autoimmune or inflammatory illnesses may lead to more severe symptoms and problems if left untreated.

Joint damage and other organ involvement are possible outcomes of untreated autoimmune disorders including rheumatoid arthritis and lupus.

6. The Development of Cancer:

Swollen lymph nodes connected to cancer, such as lymphoma or metastatic disease, may signal the spread of cancer within the body.

Delaying cancer therapy might increase the likelihood that the disease will spread to a more advanced stage, decreasing the likelihood of a successful outcome.

7. Quality of life can be negatively impacted by painful, uncomfortable lymph node swelling. Negative effects on health and productivity may result from ignoring pain and discomfort.

8. Problems in Particular Groups:

People with certain health conditions, including children, the elderly, pregnant women, and people with impaired immune systems, may be at a higher risk of problems.

Swollen glands are not always a cause for concern; in fact, many go away on their own when the underlying illness heals. However, it is essential to seek medical examination and treatment if you or someone you love develops persistent or worsening swollen glands or other troubling symptoms in order to prevent any problems and assure the best possible outcome. Addressing the underlying cause and lowering the risk of consequences depends on prompt diagnosis and treatment.

Conclusion

Enlarged glands, or lymphadenopathy, can develop from several underlying causes, including infections, inflammatory disorders, cancer, and other issues. Lymph nodes are small, bean-shaped structures that play a significant function in the immune system. When the immune system detects a threat to the body, it often responds by swelling lymph nodes.

Swollen glands can have a wide range of symptoms and associated problems, depending on the underlying reason. The area where the glands are swollen may be tender, painful, and red. Infections with bacteria and viruses, inflammatory disorders, and cancer are common triggers.

In order to treat the underlying cause of swollen glands and avoid complications, prompt identification is crucial. Depending on the underlying cause of the swelling, potential treatments may include medication, lifestyle changes, and even surgery.

Good hygiene, vaccinations, healthy lifestyle decisions, and quick treatment of diseases can all help prevent gland swelling. There may be special concerns for treating swollen glands in children, pregnant women, and those with impaired immune systems.

Infections can spread, abscesses can form, chronic illnesses can persist, and pain and discomfort can all result if swollen glands are not addressed. To get the best possible outcome and avoid complications, it is crucial to recognize the signs and seek medical assistance when necessary.

Consultation with a healthcare expert is essential for identifying the root cause of persistent or worrying symptoms connected to swollen glands and receiving suitable treatment. The illness can be better managed and subsequent consequences avoided if it is diagnosed and treated early.

THE END